CANCER CAN'T WIN

CANCER CAN'T WIN

Linda Green Rogers

To order additional copies of this book, contact:
Xlibris Corporation
1-888-795-4274
www.Xlibris.com
Orders@Xlibris.com
42131

Dedication

To all who have experienced failure and disappointment

To Thom who lived and died in a win/win situation

To God Who wants us to know the truth in II Corinthians 2:14, "But thanks be to God, who always leads us in triumph in Christ, and manifests through us the sweet aroma of the knowledge of Him."

Prologue

My Dad sat next to me and cried because he couldn't remember. I cried because I remembered. Nine months earlier my Mother died, alone, in a small Florida hospital. Dad had been in another part of the same hospital recovering from colon cancer surgery and adjusting to life ruled by Alzheimer's.

Dad and I moved back to Michigan after my husband died. A three and a half year struggle with cancer ended Thom's seven years of retirement in Florida. Now Dad and I are left, crying over memories lost and found.

"Were your Mother and I happy?" Dad asks.

I could only answer, "Yes, you were very happy."

"How long were we together?" He asks.

Patting his hand and smiling through my tears I answered, "Fifty two years."

Again he asks, "Were we happy?" And again I answer, "You were very happy."

Looking at the picture of her taken on their wedding day, Dad remarks, "She was pretty. She looks like a movie star. How did I get someone so pretty?" More tears fall.

Dad had always been so strong and intimidating. Now he's soft, broken and crying, seeking answers to simple questions concerning his life. Sometimes he looks like he's going to laugh, but instead he breaks in to a sob.

Questions continue to come. "There's a whole block of my life I can't remember. Did something terrible happen? Sometimes I wonder if I killed someone. Why can't I remember?"

Searching my face for answers he asks again, "Why can't I remember?"

I try to act nonchalant as I answer, "Dad, that just happens as we get older. It's normal." I cannot tell him, "Dad, you have Alzheimer's."

I hold back more tears watching him laboriously write names over photographs. He had taken countless pictures over the years and had neatly arranged them in albums. It was almost like he had prepared them for this time in his life. The pictures served as an anchor holding some of his memories in place.

Dad's memories of my Mother were gone, as if she never existed. Fifty-two years of marriage wiped out by Alzheimer's.

My memories tormented me. Vivid flashbacks of cancer eating away at my husband's body and tormenting his soul strutted across my mind regularly. When they took a break, images of my parents struggling with sickness, disabilities and Alzheimer's waltzed sadly by.

A lot of time has passed since that day my Dad and I cried together. He doesn't ask about my Mother anymore even though she still smiles at us from her picture setting on his dresser. My memories have lost the agony of that day, and have been replaced with a quiet sadness when one occasionally flits by.

Now I remember how God was always there giving us what we needed. I recall the many miracles and gifts of love He sent in response to our cries for help. When I thought I'd blow apart from the stress and pain God was there to give me peace and comfort. When I felt I couldn't go through another day God would wrap me in His grace.

The worse three and a half years of my life make sense only when I remember and believe what Thom continued to say throughout his battle with cancer, "I'm in a win/win situation. If I'm healed I win and if I die I win because I'll be with Jesus."

Many times it felt like we were in a lose/lose situation as our life was torn to shreds. But the truth remains, no matter how I felt or what it looked like Thom was in a win/win situation. The Bible puts it this way, "God always leads us in triumph in Christ, and manifests through us the sweet aroma of the knowledge of Him in every place" (II Corinthians 2:14).

Chapter One

"I'd rather die than move to Florida," I'd think when Thom talked of retiring there. I never said it to him, but I would act disinterested and barely reply, hoping he'd get the message. Even though he was only forty-five years old, retirement could be a reality in four years. Working for General Motors for thirty years would make a way for Thom's dream to become a reality.

His dream was to get away from Michigan's cold, dreary weather and live on a beautiful fishing lake in Florida. Thom's parents were already living out that dream and continually stirred Thom up with all their fish tales and comparisons of the warm, sunny weather they enjoyed to our nasty Michigan weather.

I tried to ignore the Florida talk hoping it would stop, but it didn't. I disliked hot, humid weather and had no desire to fish. I did not want to leave Michigan. My life was too good to give it up for fish, sweat and a state full of older retirees.

Thinking about leaving my family made me cry. I had a close relationship with my oldest daughter Heather and couldn't bear the thought of leaving her. She and her husband Todd had been married five years and were talking about having a baby. What kind of grandmother could I be living twelve hundred miles away? When I'd see my sister enjoy her grandchildren, I'd be tormented with sadness knowing I wouldn't have that closeness with mine if I lived in Florida.

Then I'd think about my parents and cry more. My Mother had suffered a stroke leaving her unable to care for herself. My Dad, who had never done a bit of housework, had to learn to cook, clean, do laundry, and take care of my Mother. Every week I'd cook them a meal, do a bit of cleaning, and take Mom out for lunch and shopping. I tried to lighten their load and bring some pleasure into their lives.

It was a terrible situation for my parents to deal with, but it brought a closeness to my family we'd never experienced. For the first time I saw my Dad truly care for my Mom and heard her call him, "Sweetheart." Hugging and saying, "I love you," became normal for us after forty some years of keeping our distance. Praying together replaced our past disagreements over what we believed God was all about.

How could I think of moving twelve hundred miles away? Who would be there for my daughter and parents? How could I get along without them close by?

I had the greatest friends anyone could have. We started out twenty years earlier as young families raising our children together. We attended the same church and helped each other through the storms of life we each faced. They knew everything about me and my family and still loved us unconditionally. It had taken many years of exposing our true selves to each other to build the solid relationships we shared. I knew I could never be a part of something so deep and genuine again. How could I make a move across the country?

Church played a major role in our lives, and we belonged to one of the best in the state. I taught classes at the Bible Training Institute when it first began. I watched it grow into an accredited Bible school, and I had a part in preparing many aspiring ministers. My passion was teaching the Word of God. I was established as a credible teacher and given the privilege to teach as much as I wanted. It was my dream come true and I couldn't bear the thought of giving it up.

Perfect life? I thought it was as perfect as life could be for me. Even my part-time job as a hairdresser in a nursing home often seemed too good to be true. I worked two days a week and made as much in those two days as others made in a week. The nursing home had just built me a new shop that made my work even more enjoyable. That job seemed to be a once-in-a-lifetime deal. I was certain I couldn't find anything comparable in Florida.

My roots went deep-winding around family, friends, church, ministry, job and home. I was born, raised, married, and living my life all within a five-mile radius. Lansing, Michigan, was my home. I loved my life, and I did not want to be uprooted and planted twelve hundred miles away.

While visiting my in-laws at their fishing haven in Florida, Thom began to talk seriously about moving down. I could no longer act disinterested and hope he'd forget it. I was being hit head-on with his dream.

Depression gripped me and all I wanted to do was cry. Then anger would set in, and I wanted to scream at him, "Are you nuts? Why would you want to leave all we have in Michigan to come down here? I hate this place!" However, I kept quiet and struggled.

Unable to sleep one night, I shut myself in the closet and let the tears flow, muffling my sobs with a pillow. I cried out to God in my desperation, "Help me! What am I going to do? You know I can't stand the idea of moving to this hot, humid place. I hate Florida! I'd rather die than live here!"

When I finally quieted down, I heard His answer loud and clear. From deep within my heart came God's answer to my plea.

"You help Thom fulfill his dream, and I'll take care of yours." Short and simple, God had spoken. I didn't cry or argue, instead I said, "Okay Lord, I'll obey You."

Peace washed over me followed by relief that the struggle was over. I felt an excitement for this new adventure begin to rise up within me.

Looking back over the years, I'm so thankful God answered my cry for help and gave me direction. It wasn't my way, but God knows our lives from beginning to end. He often leads in ways we don't understand until much later. He has the whole picture while we only see part of it. I could have chosen to disobey and have my own way and Thom would not have had his dream fulfilled.

Obedience to God or disobedience effects more people than we can imagine. Failing to obey God hurts many people. Adam is a prime example, the whole human race suffered for his one act of disobedience. "For as through the one man's disobedience the many were made sinners" (Romans 5:19). How many people will suffer when we choose to disobey God?

Choosing to obey God also touches many people in good ways. The obedience of Jesus turned around the whole mess that Adam started when he chose to do what he wanted rather than what God wanted. "Even so through the obedience of the One the many will be made righteous" (Romans 5:19).

When God is dealing with us about doing something His way or our own way we must think about the great number of people that will be affected by our decision. Obedience to God always has a positive effect bringing life and blessings. Disobedience brings destruction and death. Isaiah 1:19-20 says, "If you consent and obey, you will eat the best of the land; but if you refuse and rebel, you will be devoured by the sword."

Chapter Two

Less than twenty-four hours after letting go of my way and choosing to obey God, Thom and I found ourselves sitting in the home of our future neighbor. Oddly enough, he was a realtor.

We had gone for a walk in his parent's neighborhood enjoying the beauty of the night. The orange and grapefruit trees were loaded with fruit and palm trees graced every yard. The air was balmy with a soft breeze. The sound of a distant alligator grunting and the hooting of an owl gave the night a special feel.

That night I began the conversation about moving to Florida. If Thom was surprised, he didn't show it but joined in excitedly talking about how beautiful it was right there in that neighborhood. Nearing the end of the street, we noticed a cute little house for sale. It was empty, so we began peeking in the windows. We didn't get to look much before the neighbor's lights came on, and a man stepped outside asking, "Can I help you folks?"

Thom, who never met a stranger, started telling him his dream of retiring and moving to Florida.

"I'm Bill, and I'm a realtor. Why don't you come in and tell me more about what you are looking for."

Bill and his wife had moved to Lake Wales several years ago from New York. A kind man and distinguished looking in his early seventies, Bill immediately gained our confidence.

After listening to our plan Bill advised us against buying a house. He suggested we buy a lot that we could build on when the time came for us to move. He just happened to have a lot available on the next street, so we set up an appointment to see it the next day.

I voiced my biggest concern to Bill, "What about churches? We'll be leaving a great one in Michigan, and we have to have a good church to be a part of."

I told him about my involvement in ministry and what we wanted in a church. The next day the pastor from the First Assembly of God Church in

Lake Wales called us at Thom's parents' home informing us that Bill had told him about us. After Thom and the pastor talked, we knew First Assembly would one day be our new church home.

As soon as we saw the lot we knew it was the one for us. The price was right, and the location seemed perfect. It was on a canal that flowed into Lake Pierce, a popular fishing lake well-known for prize-winning bass. The lot was big enough to build the type of house we wanted, and it was cleared and ready for action. Six months later the lot was ours.

It continued to be more obvious that God's plan for us was to move to Florida where Thom's dream would become a reality. Every step we took toward the move seemed orchestrated from above. I never again thought, "I'd rather die than move to Florida." I still felt sad that I would have to leave my daughter and parents, friends and church, but I also felt an excitement about this new life God was leading us to.

Holly, our youngest daughter, made the move with us. She hadn't been happy and didn't know what she wanted to do with her life. Moving to Florida with new possibilities to explore looked good to our twenty-year-old. Now she claims Florida as her home and vows never to live in Michigan again.

When I look back, I thank God He spoke to my heart that night I cried out to him from the closet and that I chose to obey. I'll never forget His words to me, "You help Thom fulfill his dream, and I'll take care of yours." Short, simple, and doable, that's how God leads us. He never tells us to do something without supplying all the tools needed to complete the job. Thoughts, feelings and practicalities, God took care of them all.

Selling our home was hard on my emotions. We had lived there all of our married life, twenty-six years. We loved our home. We watched it being built, we laid the sod, we planted trees, and we watched neighbors move in and out. Our two daughters grew up there; the house was filled with memories. Many friends and family had filled the house enjoying parties, Bible studies, my beauty shop in the basement, and just hanging out. It had been the perfect house for us, but the time came to leave it and move on to another perfect house.

We didn't have to look at many floor plans before we found the one we both liked. Getting the right builder could have been a challenge, but God had one lined up for us. After a couple phone calls we knew we'd found the right one even though there was twelve-hundred miles between us. When the completed floor plans arrived from him the first thing we saw printed in the corner was Psalm 127:1. We grabbed the Bible and read, "Unless the Lord builds the house, they labor in vain who build it."

Our house sold within a few months, but the trailer on the lake was at a standstill, and time was running out. Thom loved to go fishing at night, often staying out until sunrise. On the last Saturday of August, at midnight, he was out fishing and talking to the Lord. Thinking he was alone on the lake, he said out aloud, "Lord, You know we've got to sell this trailer before we can move, but no one is interested in buying it. What are we going to do? I give up."

A voice called out from the dark shadows of the lake, "Is somebody there? Can I help you?"

The sound of oars plowing through the water preceded the boat that came up alongside of Thom's boat, and a young man asked, "Was that you I heard talking?"

"Well, I was talking to God," Thom told the man. He then shared his dream of retiring and moving to Florida and that he needed the trailer to sell.

"I'm a Christian," he told Thom, "I'd like to pray with you about this."

The two of them prayed that God would send someone to buy the trailer within the week. It was 12:30 a.m. Sunday. At 12:30 p.m. that same Sunday a couple looked at the trailer and bought it. Again God made a way.

When God tells us to do something He always makes a way for us to do it. He will take care of all the details that can overwhelm us. Remember how He took care of His people when they left Egypt. He provided food from heaven, water gushed out of the rocks for them to drink, their shoes didn't wear out and none of them were sick or feeble. He even split the Red Sea for them to pass through and escape the Egyptians pursuing them. God will open our Red Seas and pour out on us abilities and supplies to complete what He has told us to do.

Moving into our custom built house on the lake was the beginning of Thom's dream coming true. I'd never seen him so happy. His tedious factory job was history and no more cold, wet, unpredictable Michigan weather to bear. Thom was a free man, free to bask in the Florida sun by day and fish for the "big one" late into the night or before the sun came up in the morning.

It would have been enough for me to see Thom enjoying life, but God promised He would take care of my dream too. A week after arriving in Florida, I started a job as a writer for the town's weekly newspaper.

Working for the eighty-year-old owner of a small town paper was like taking a wonderful trip back in time. I pounded out obituaries, wedding stories, and local news on a typewriter that could have been sold as an antique. I learned the town's local history only a small town newspaper staff would know and remember. After six months of being a newspaper reporter, I got bored with writing obituaries and weddings. The "snowbirds" had gone north for the summer leaving little news to report. I realized I didn't have what it takes to go prying for a good story, so I quit.

My next six-month adventure was learning rental property management and secretarial duties in a local real estate office. I soon tired of the mundane office tasks and trying to fill my eight-hour days looking busy.

When I complained to the Lord, I felt Him directing me to hang on until January; it was then October. I missed working in a beauty shop helping women feel better about themselves while creating flattering hairstyles. What I didn't know at the time was that God was preparing a place for me at a beauty shop in a retirement community. In December I saw an ad for a hairdresser; I applied and was hired and began working in January.

Within a few months I was asked to manage the shop. I accepted and began the challenge of rebuilding a failing business. It was great fun trusting God to bring the right help, draw customers to the shop and equip us to give the women the best hairdos they'd ever had. It was even more fun and exciting to see God open doors for me to teach a Bible study at the shop and to pray for the customers that shared their problems. On top of all that, I was making more money than I'd ever made.

We were experiencing the truth of God's Word, "If you consent and obey, you will eat the best of the land" (Isaiah 1:19). Obeying God always brings the best. It may hurt a bit to give up our desires to do what He says to do, but it will always turn out for our good.

Thom began his work adventures a few months after moving in and getting the house and yard finished. He, too, had a couple short-term jobs before finding the place he would be happy and fulfilled.

Building screen porches he got to know all the back roads in the county and enjoyed his friendship with his job partner. Then he landed a job, quite unexpectedly, at a local car dealership as a quality control representative. After six months they fired him because of a disagreement about company policies.

Shocked, embarrassed, and sad at losing his job, Thom was sure nothing could compare to the impressive position he'd held. But God had everything in place for the greatest work experience of his life.

A friend at church told him about an opening at the golf shop in a private and exclusive community where he worked as a guard at the front gate. Thom applied for the job and got hired, even though he never played golf and knew nothing about the game.

Friendly and hard-working, he soon fit in at the golf shop. Most of the residents were retired and Thom went out of his way to serve them and treat them with respect and kindness. He loved the people there and they loved him.

Losing his job at the dealership seemed like a blow, but God had something so much better for Thom. The four years he spent working there were the most enjoyable years of his life. He felt good about himself and knew the people loved and respected him-something he had missed out on working thirty-one years in a car factory.

When the shop closed in the summer, he worked on the greens, mowing and planting flowers. Thom's roots grew deep in the soil of that community, both in the ground and in the hearts of the people.

Jeremiah 29:11 was a reality for us. "For I know the plans I have for you, declares the Lord, plans for welfare (shalom: completeness, soundness, peace) and not for calamity, to give you a future and a hope." We would have missed out on being made complete and sound if I had continued to want my own way, refusing to move to Florida.

Our daughter, Holly, also experienced the goodness of God's plans for her. She began her adventure working in a daycare while getting an associate's degree at the community college. She worked for the school board and a couple years later went to work for the sheriff's department where she met her husband and is living "happily ever-after."

A year after we moved my parents bought a new home six miles away and joined us in Florida. My mother wasn't too happy about pulling up her roots that had been growing in Michigan for eighty years but I believe she enjoyed our times together and the sunny weather. Dad loved everything about Florida, especially being able to be outside all year with no bad weather to contend with. Of course I was ecstatic to have them close by and knew it was another gift from God for my obedience to Him.

About every four months I spent time with my oldest daughter and her husband. When the grandchildren, Rebecca and Bailey, came I made sure they knew who their Nana was. God provided for us to keep our relationships close and special.

Life was good in Florida. God was blessing us more than we'd ever experienced. We were satisfied in our church, we had wonderful new friends, we loved our jobs, we kept our family close and we had a blast living in Florida.

Chapter Three

Our fourth summer in Florida was full of good times except for a tiny suspicion that something wasn't quite right. I tried to ignore it and Thom denied it.

He was enjoying himself working on the long-awaited seawall, fishing late nights and early mornings, working a few days a week on the golf course, and serving as a deacon at church. Life had never been so full and pleasurable for Thom. He was doing everything he loved to do. The only thing missing to complete the dream was for Heather, Todd and new granddaughter Rebecca to live in Florida too.

Life was a joy except for that tiny, nagging suspicion that something wasn't right. The feeling grew when we spent a few days with Heather, Todd and Rebecca at Vero Beach. We played in the pool with our toddling granddaughter and dipped her tiny toes in the ocean waves. We enjoyed seafood and steaks at the Patio and ice cream at Swenson's.

I'd look at my beautiful family and almost burst with joy and thankfulness that God would bless me so much. Then I'd catch a glimpse of Thom and see pain, or was it worry, on his face. I noticed him taking aspirin quite often which was extremely unusual for a man that absolutely refused to take one for a headache. Now he seemed to be taking them regularly.

Many times over the summer I asked him, "What's wrong? Why are you taking so many aspirin?"

He'd never give me an answer. I'd threaten to make a doctor's appointment for him, but he always replied vehemently, "I won't go!"

Guilt still tries to harass me, whispering in my ear, "If you had called a doctor things would have turned out differently."

I try to excuse myself with, "We didn't have a family doctor, and besides, I didn't know what I'd tell them Thom needed to be there for. And he wouldn't have gone."

I should have found a doctor and made an appointment and did everything in my power to get him there. But God . . . I've come to depend on the "But Gods" in my life. But God is so much bigger than all my mistakes. Even the mistake of not taking Thom's twenty-five-pound weight loss over the summer as a blaring signal that something was wrong. I thought it was from all the hard work he'd done on the seawall in the hot sun. He'd always been one to lose weight quickly and easily.

By the end of summer I was getting pretty nervous about the things I'd been seeing. They weren't going away as I had hoped they would. I got up the nerve to ask my daughter that had been down for a visit if she noticed anything wrong. She couldn't pinpoint anything and assured me, "Dad is fine." Certainly if she didn't notice anything then nothing could be wrong I reasoned.

It seemed like other people would have noticed if something was wrong. Especially his mother who could find things wrong that weren't wrong.

We were a family that hated confrontation or anything that would disrupt our peace. Our secret motto was "Peace at any price." It was so much easier to pretend everything was okay, to pretend the suspicions had no ground to stand on.

Peace is good, but sometimes we need to make waves, confront, step out, and do what is uncomfortable for us. Jesus didn't always bring peace into situations. He stirred people up at times when they needed stirring up. How many people would have missed out on meeting Jesus if He had not confronted the woman at the well? What if He had thought, "Well, I don't want to make her mad or upset by telling her she has had five husbands and the one she is now living with isn't her husband." When Jesus confronted her she went back to town and told everyone she had found the Messiah. Jesus stayed there for two days teaching them about the kingdom of God and many believed in Him (John 4:7-43).

Remember the man that had been ill for thirty-eight years and waited by the pool of Bethesda, hoping to be the first to get in and be healed? Jesus approached him and asked, "Do you wish to get well?" (John 5:6) He was bold and got right to the root of the problem. I can't believe it was comfortable asking him if he wanted to get well but the man got healed when Jesus confronted him with the truth.

Fear is a deceiver. It whispers, "It's nothing; ignore it, and it will go away." Sometimes we deceive ourselves into thinking that we trust God by ignoring a problem. Faith comes when we expose the problem, and seek God for the solution.

Fear will drive us so far from the problem that it appears to be too late when we finally do face it. It is never too late for God to make right a bad situation.

I believe God always prepares us for an upcoming battle but we often don't listen or pay attention to His warnings. Early in the spring, we received a letter from a friend in Tennessee. Ella had been a neighbor and later became part of the women's ministry I directed. She had been a close friend and prayer partner. We kept in touch with a Christmas letter, so I was surprised to hear from her in the spring.

Her letter described in great detail a dream she had about Thom. He was in a fight with a huge, strong giant of a man. They fought and fought, knocking a table and chairs over. Thom got hit hard several times but kept fighting. The dream had no ending, just fighting and struggling. Ella said she was interceding for Thom and felt we should know about the dream.

I tried to figure it out. I was certain it concerned smoking, a problem Thom still hadn't dealt with even after promises to quit when we moved to Florida. Now, looking back, I see it was God warning us, wanting to prepare us for the battle that was to come. I don't know if Thom took Ella's dream seriously. I knew it was from God and I did pray but after a few weeks I forgot about it.

April is the most beautiful month in Florida; it's not too hot, and everything is in full bloom. Driving to work one morning I was enjoying the warm air blowing on my face, smelling flowers in the air and feeling full of peace and contentment. Suddenly I was hit with a blow to my heart as I distinctly heard these words, "This sickness is not unto death but for the glory of God."

I knew God had dropped that verse into my heart from the eleventh chapter of the Gospel of John. I remembered that Jesus had said this to His disciples when He got word that Lazarus was very sick. Lazarus did die, but Jesus raised him from the dead after being in the tomb four days.

My first thought was, "Oh no, am I going to get sick? God, what does this mean?"

I knew it was God speaking to me. I couldn't ignore it or forget it. I had no idea what those words, "this sickness is not unto death but for the glory of God," were going to mean to me. I only knew I must not take them lightly.

Chapter Four

Summer ended, the snowbirds returned and we were happy to get back into our busy work schedules. We looked forward to the evenings telling each other the news about who we'd seen that day. The retired people I took care of at the beauty shop and the ones Thom served in the golf shop had become an important part of our lives. We loved hearing about their families, listening to their troubles, and rejoicing with them when they played a good golf game, won at bingo or got word their family was coming to visit.

Our full days helped us forget about Thom's weight loss and continual need for aspirin. It all came crashing in on me the night I was cutting Thom's hair. When I bent down to trim the left side I saw it, a lump the size of a quarter, just below his ear and in line with his jaw. I couldn't believe what I was seeing. How long had it been there? Why hadn't I seen it before?

Instantly my stomach got sick, my body felt numb and all I could think was, "What am I going to do?"

Fear wrapped its ugly tentacles around me and began to squeeze so tight I could hardly breathe. I continued to cut his hair trying to act normal. I couldn't get past the thought, "What am I going to do?"

Quickly and quietly I finished the haircut, swept the hair and put the scissors and comb away. Thom returned to watching television and I hurried to my office where I often spent time. I turned on the desk lamp, laid out my Bible and paper to look like I was preparing for Sunday's lesson and buried my face in my arms.

Now I had to do something even though everything in me wanted to pretend I didn't see the lump. The suspicions I'd had for the past five months all came rushing back to taunt me. Fear and denial had ruled me then. Now the fear of what the lump meant began to choke me. Knowing I had to confront Thom made me sick with dread.

All I could do was cry out, "Lord, what am I going to do? What am I going to do? Oh, God, what am I going to do?"

I didn't do anything for the next few days except pray. I didn't talk to anyone about it. I just prayed and waited. I had to hear from God. I had to get strong. I could not handle this one on my own.

Every Monday I got together to pray with Karen, her mother Mildred, Robin and Cathy. God had knit our hearts together over the past several months as we prayed for each other and the struggling church where we had met. When I left Michigan I thought I'd never find the kind of extraordinary friends I'd left there but God had it all planned out. These four women had become the friends I would so desperately need.

I sat quietly for some time, listening to the others talk. Finally I blurted out the terrible secret I'd been carrying the past few days. I told them the suspicions I'd had and Thom's refusal to talk. I ended it sobbing, "What am I going to do?"

I felt their love envelop me and peace began to replace the fear that had been so overpowering. Before they said a word my load began to lighten and I knew what Paul was talking about when he said, "Bear one another's burdens" (Galatians 6:2).

Karen responded first, "You've got to talk to Thom about it." I knew that would have to be done tonight. Before the fear could grab me again she lovingly gave me the encouragement I needed.

"Oh, Linda," Cathy's voice was full of compassion, "we're going to pray for Thom. God will heal him." She had experienced God's miracles many times and this was another opportunity to see God work.

Always looking for ways to help others, Robin said, "We're here for you and Thom. We'll do anything we can to help." Over the next four years Robin remained our steadfast and committed friend, doing whatever she could to lighten our load.

Then Mildred shared her experience of having tongue cancer. I didn't know that was what caused the slight droop on one side of her mouth. She told me about the wonderful and kind doctor that had done her surgery. Mostly she praised God for helping her through it and healing her.

Mildred finished by saying, "My doctor has an office in town. You must make an appointment for Thom right away."

For the past several days my only prayer had been, "What am I going to do?" Now I had my answer. I would talk to Thom that night. I would pray and trust God to heal him. I would make an appointment with Mildred's doctor immediately. I would let our friends help us.

Karen, Mildred, Robin and Cathy gathered around me and prayed. It seemed like God and all His angels filled Cathy's little house in Dundee,

Florida that day. He removed the fear that had me paralyzed. He gave me the strength to face the problem head on. He assured me that all would be well.

Friends are from God, gifts to be treasured. Each one has a something to give, words to comfort and encourage, prayers to pray, and love to share. At times life can be so hard but a friend can instantly bring the love of God into the situation. I learned how desperately we need each other. I thank God for all the incredible friends He has always provided for me.

I cried all the way home from Cathy's house. I cried tears of relief that my dreaded secret was out. I cried tears of gratitude that God had prepared such special friends for me. Mostly I cried for Thom.

After a quiet supper I knew the time had come for me to confront Thom. I'd spent the afternoon praying but I still didn't feel ready but I'd probably never feel ready for what I had to face.

I decided to jump right in, "Thom we need to talk."

He always hated to hear those words because it usually meant we were in for an explosive argument. There would be no fighting tonight.

I continued, "The other night when I was cutting your hair I saw a big lump on your neck. How long has that been there? What's going on?"

I'm sure he was as relieved as I was to get this awful secret out in the open. He told me about the sores and pain in his tongue that had plagued him all summer and now into the fall.

"That's why you were taking so much aspirin." I started to cry. "Why didn't you tell me?"

"My Grandpa had tongue cancer," he explained. "They cut part of his tongue out and he sat around and drooled until he died. I didn't want to be like that."

Even though that had been forty years earlier those memories had tied Thom up with fear, preventing him from getting medical help in the early stage of cancer. Fear is a wicked thing that has to be faced and pushed out of our way. The Bible tells us three hundred and sixty six times, in different ways, to not fear, once for every day of the year, including leap year.

I told him about our friend Mildred, "She had tongue cancer seven years ago and you'd never know it now. They can do so much more now than when your grandpa had it. Mildred's doctor has an office in Lake Wales and she said he is the best. Can I call for an appointment for you?"

"I guess I have to do something don't I? Yes, go ahead and make an appointment." I saw the same relief come over Thom that I'd felt earlier that day after sharing with my friends.

"Oh Thom, we've seen God do so many miracles. I know He is going to heal you. Want to pray together right now?" Holding hands we went before God with our mountain of trouble.

We hadn't developed a consistent prayer life together as a couple. We had gone our separate ways spiritually, doing our own thing with God. What a huge mistake husbands and wives make by not praying together every day. The power that is available to a married couple in unity is unlimited. Jesus said in Matthew 18:19, "Again I say to you, that if two of you agree on earth about anything that they may ask, it shall be done for them by My Father who is in heaven."

Chapter Five

Tuesday morning I called the doctor. He could see Thom on Thursday afternoon. I couldn't wait to get there and find out what the doctor had to say about Thom's condition. Then I'd be filled with dread, not wanting to hear his diagnosis.

I rearranged my afternoon appointments at the beauty shop and Thom had the day off. We tried to be cheerful and positive as we headed for town but I felt as cold, dark and dreary as the weather was that day. It seemed like the sun disappeared from the universe, reflecting how I felt.

After filling out all the necessary papers we settled down to wait our turn. There were several others waiting and one of the women looked familiar to me. She caught me looking at her and said, "You look familiar. Where do I know you from?"

"I think I've seen you at church," I replied.

"Oh yes," she said, "that's it. So what are you two doing here?"

We anxiously shared the reason for being there. She immediately responded, "Can I pray for you?"

All I could say was, "Please do." I didn't care that the waiting room was full. The three of us grabbed hands and she began to pray.

"Oh Lord, we come to You in the mighty name of Jesus, I ask you to fill these two with Your peace, peace that passes all understanding. I ask You to give them the strength they need to face this problem. I ask you to give the doctor wisdom, show him what to do, how to care for Thom. I thank You that You have provided healing, that Jesus bore Thom's pains and carried his sickness and that by Your stripes he is healed according to Isaiah 53. Please surround them with Your love and lead them by Your Spirit, In Jesus name, Amen."

I felt like God Himself had set up this time of prayer for us. He had appointed this woman to be there when we were in desperate need.

The horrible dread I'd come in with was gone, replaced with peace. I knew we could get through this and God would lead us every step of the way. Thom had a calmness about him that hadn't been there when we arrived.

We barely had time to tell her how much she had ministered to us and how grateful we were that she would be bold enough to pray for us there. The nurse was calling, "Thomas Green, you can come with me," as we said our final "thank you."

The doctor looked and probed and x-rayed Thom's mouth and neck. I didn't like the grave look on his face or the lack of conversation. When he finished the exam he painted a very serious picture of what was going on.

He was blunt and didn't try to soften the blow saying, "It is cancer. It has traveled from the tongue and wrapped around the carotid artery. Surgery can be done but if it is too close to the artery it can't be removed. Part of the tongue will have to be taken off. I'd like to set you up with my partner and he will do the surgery."

My heart was breaking for Thom. This report was worse than anything I could have imagined. How could this be happening to us? I looked at Thom and couldn't believe how calm he appeared.

I got myself to the waiting room while Thom took care of business with the office girl. I sat next to a pretty young woman and her husband. When Thom came out the man asked, "Are you okay?"

Thom told him, "No," and shared what the doctor had said.

The couple listened attentively and responded with compassion, "Can we pray with you?"

For the second time that afternoon we were desperate for help and again, God had appointed someone to be there to pray with us. The four of us stood together, holding hands, oblivious to the other people.

Both husband and wife prayed for us asking God for healing, strength, comfort and help. They didn't end their prayer with "if it be Thy will," but "By His stripes Thom was healed" (Isaiah 53:4). This couple knew it was God's will to heal Thom and that Jesus had taken all his pain and sickness on His own body at the cross. They knew the authority Jesus had given all believers and commanded the cancer to go from his body. (Luke 10:19, Mark 16:18)

What a gift of love we received from three strangers that dreadful day in the doctor's office. It cost them nothing but the risk that we'd refuse their offer and they would be embarrassed for asking if they could pray for us. Their prayers that day were priceless treasures to us, costing nothing but valued beyond any monetary gift we could have received. How many times have we missed opportunities to give priceless gifts of prayer to the people we meet every day?

The next hurdle we had to jump was telling our family what we were facing. Thom's parents would be the hardest. Ma tended to be emotional and often blurted out whatever she thought and felt. Pa had always claimed to be an atheist and didn't need God.

The past thirty years they had pestered Thom about his smoking habit. When we moved to Florida they made an offer, which he declined, to pay for a hypnotist to help him quit. We were sure their response to our news would be, "We tried to tell you." Instead they quietly listened as we explained the details of our visit to the doctor.

"Oh, Tommy," Ma cried, "it's just like my Dad."

I quickly jumped in with, "but that was forty years ago, they can do so much more now. And we know that God is healing Thom."

Then Thom stepped in and confidently said, "I'm in a win/win situation. If I'm healed I win and if I die and go to heaven I win. I can't lose no matter what happens."

Thom's statement settled over us like a giant cloud of peace. No one had any thing to say so Thom asked, "can we pray together?"

I knew Ma would not have a problem with praying but Pa might put up a fuss. He had always been so strong about not believing in God.

We were about to receive our third gift of love that day as they both answered with a soft but determined, "Yes."

I'd been part of this family for over thirty years. That night, for the first time, as we prayed for Thom's healing our hearts were knit together in love and unity. Thom was deeply touched to have his parents pray with him and for him. It was a gift of love that would last forever.

Another gift came the next day when Thom's mother told us she had forgiven her brother in law. She had hated him for forty-five years and blamed him for her sister's tragic death. I'd talked to her several months before about forgiving him but she insisted she never could. Not only did she get set free from the bondage of unforgiveness but she expressed her desire to surrender control of her life to Jesus. I had the privilege of praying with her to receive Jesus Christ as her Lord and Savior.

We took another bold step and asked them to come to church with us the following Sunday. Ma quickly said, "Yes." Pa hesitated and said, "I'll let you know."

Thom's parents did come to church with us. We were elated and a bit apprehensive. Anything could happen at our charismatic church and that day it was unusually spirited. At the door Pa reminded us, "Now that I'm here the roof will probably fall in."

The worship leader was a young man, maybe twenty years old and full of enthusiasm. The music was loud and lively. Halfway through the second song there was a glitch in the sound equipment. It sounded like a bolt of lightning striking the church. It was so loud we could feel the vibrations. It seemed like the roof was falling in.

Next the pastor told the congregation, "Brother Thom has been diagnosed with cancer and is scheduled for surgery Tuesday morning. Brother Thom, please come up here so we can pray for you."

Thom went forward and shared with the church, "I'm in a win/win situation. If I'm healed I win and if I die I win because I'll be in heaven with Jesus."

Pastor asked everyone to stretch their hands out toward Thom and pray. I sneaked a peek at Ma and Pa; their hands were stretched out too. Everyone around us was praying in tongues, loudly binding the devil in Jesus name or shouting, "Hallelujah."

I prayed for Ma and Pa, "Oh Lord, help them to see You and not be shocked." Neither of them had ever been in a charismatic church. They were seeing and hearing things foreign to their church experience.

After several minutes of intense prayer the pastor and several others laid hands on Thom praying for healing according to Mark 16:17-18. "These signs will accompany those who have believed: in My name they will cast out demons, they will speak with new tongues; they will pick up serpents, and if they drink any deadly poison, it will not hurt them; they will lay hands on the sick, and they will recover."

Sitting down I thought, "Now things will settle down." As I looked up there towered in front of us a thin man with long hair and a beard. He had been sitting a few rows behind us.

"I have a word for you, Brother Thom." He began encouraging him with words from the Bible. I could feel a powerful presence, the anointing of God. Everyone seemed to be holding their breath waiting for each word to be spoken.

When he finished speaking he toppled over backward like a giant tree being cut down. He didn't crumple at the knees, but went straight back and down with no one to break his fall. There had to be an angel there to ease him down because he didn't flinch or make a sound when he hit the floor.

I wasn't surprised to see him fall down under the power of God; I felt weak and shaky and glad I was sitting down. I didn't know how I'd explain it to Ma and Pa. I was certain they had never seen this happen before even though it was quite common in charismatic services. I decided if they didn't ask I'd leave it alone and let God take care of them.

When the service ended we thanked them for coming and tried to express how much it meant to us that they were there. It was a gift of love we would be eternally grateful for.

Chapter Six

Thom's surgery was to take place the Tuesday before Thanksgiving. He always enjoyed getting together with his family and eating lots of turkey, stuffing and all the fixings. This holiday he would only have a liquid supplement poured directly into his stomach through a feeding tube.

We left for the hospital at 5:30 a.m. We tried to be lighthearted but heaviness hung over us. Thom had always been so healthy. What were we doing in this predicament? Hospitals and doctors had no place in our lives. Pulling in to the hospital parking lot my only thought was, "We don't belong here."

I was glad when they sedated Thom. I couldn't bear to see him laying on the gurney looking so vulnerable. The doctor's words came taunting me, "Its cancer." My mind shouted, "Thom's going to die!"

Whispering in my heart God shut out those murderous voices and said, "Don't be afraid. Trust Me."

"How can I? This is too awful."

Again the still, small voice strongly answered, "You will do it step by step, day by day for I am the One in control."

I thought I knew how to trust God. I'd trusted Him for everything life had thrown at me but cancer was the thing I dreaded more than anything. When I saw others deal with cancer I'd think, "I could not go through that, please God, don't ever let me have to." I wanted no part of such a destructive monster, but then, who does?

I had to continually remind myself of the promise God had given me, "This sickness is not unto death but for the glory of God" (John 11:4). Tormenting thoughts were always ready to fill my mind so I had to constantly choose to think about God's Word.

When I first became a Christian I was excited to learn that God is a good God, that He loves me and only wants the best for me. I'd always heard things like, "God punishes us," or "God teaches us by putting bad stuff on us."

Studying the Bible I learned that sickness is not from God but from the devil. "Your adversary, the devil, prowls around like a roaring lion, seeking someone to devour. But resist him, firm in your faith, knowing that the same experiences of suffering are being accomplished by your brethren who are in the world" (I Peter 5:8-9).

My excitement grew when I read in Matthew 8:16-17 that Jesus healed them all and "this was to fulfill what was spoken through Isaiah the prophet: HE HIMSELF TOOK OUR INFIRMITIES AND CARRIED AWAY OUR DISEASES." When I looked for what the prophet Isaiah foretold I found it in Isaiah 53:4-5. "Surely our griefs (the Hebrew word is choli which means sickness) He Himself bore, and our sorrows (the Hebrew word is makob which means pains) He carried; yet we ourselves esteemed Him stricken, smitten of God, and afflicted. But He was pierced through for our transgressions, He was crushed for our iniquities; the chastening for our well-being fell upon Him, and by His scourging we were healed."

Jesus took care of our sins. He was punished for us. Jesus got to the root of sickness which is sin. He took on His own body all of our sin and sickness, sickness in our body and our soul which is our mind, will and emotions.

I had learned the truth about sickness and healing many years before and now I was facing the real deal. Did I really believe what I had read in the Bible? Was I ready to do what I had told others to do when they faced sickness? Could I believe God's Word no matter what the doctors said? Could I believe God's Word no matter what I saw taking place in Thom's body?

When Jesus healed He often said things like, "Your faith has made you well," (Matthew 9:22) or "It shall be done to you according to your faith" (Matthew 9:29). He said He couldn't do many miracles in His hometown because of their unbelief (Matthew 13:58). He often chided His disciples for their lack or littleness of faith. The disciples were unable to drive out a demon and asked Jesus why. He told them, "Because of the littleness of your faith; for truly I say to you, if you have faith the size of a mustard seed, you will say to this mountain, 'Move from here to there,' and it will move; and nothing will be impossible to you" (Matthew 17:20).

Thom and I knew all these things. We had gone to churches that taught the truth about healing. We had experienced many miracles during the past twenty five years. Our daughter had been miraculously healed of anorexia. Thom had been delivered from alcoholism by the power of God. Two of our closest friends were totally healed of lupus and cancer. We had been born again, forgiven of all our sins and made brand new creations. God Himself lived in us. How could we not believe Thom would be healed of cancer?

Thom's faith was in God's promise that no matter what hit him in this life he is a winner. That is why he continued to say, "I'm in a win/win situation." He believed Romans 8:37-39, "But in all these things we overwhelmingly conquer through Him who loved us. For I am convinced that neither death, nor life, nor angels, nor principalities, nor things present, nor things to come, nor powers, nor height, nor depth, nor any other created thing, will be able to separate us from the love of God, which is in Christ Jesus our Lord."

Three hours passed before the doctor came to the surgical waiting room. I searched his face for signs of success. I didn't like the serious look he had on his face. I wanted him to come in smiling and say, "It was much less than I thought and we were able to remove every bit of cancer. He will be back to normal in no time."

Instead he went into great detail, most of which I didn't comprehend. I only wanted to hear good news so I asked him, "Can I be happy about the surgery?" He replied, "Yes."

The next day when I got to the hospital Thom was sitting up, alert and happy. We were told he would be unable to talk for quite some time because his tongue would be so swollen and painful. I was shocked and elated when he answered my question, "How are you doing?"

He was so excited telling me how he startled the doctor early that morning. While he was reviewing Thom's chart and preparing to examine him Thom said, "Good morning, Doctor. How are you?" He took great delight in the look of shock the doctor gave him as he responded to his patient's supernatural progress, "You aren't supposed to be able to talk yet."

Always quick with an answer, Thom told him, "God had a better idea."

Thanksgiving was spent in the hospital but Thom didn't care. Even the feeding tube in his stomach didn't seem to bother him. When I arrived Thursday morning he was bubbling over about one of the gentleman he took care of at the golf shop. He had brought a can of sardines with a note saying, "Paid in full for your service." Thom had done him a favor and when the man asked him, "What do I owe you," Thom told him, "A can of sardines." That can of sardines meant more to Thom than all the flowers in Florida. If only we knew the profound effect we can have on others by a simple act of kindness.

Thom's recovery was quick. Within a few weeks he was back to work at the golf shop telling everyone about the goodness of God and the can of sardines. He had always been bold about his faith in God and now he had a healing testimony to share and he did.

Chapter Seven

The Friday before Christmas Thom was scheduled to meet with the doctor that would be in charge of his radiation treatments. He emphasized the need to begin treatments as soon as possible to stop the growth of any cancer cells the surgeon may have missed.

Precise measurements were taken of Thom's mouth, face and neck. A heavy plaster mask was made to protect the portion of his head and face that didn't need radiation. They picked and probed, took blood and asked every imaginable question. We both were overwhelmed, nervous and exhausted when the doctor hit us with the last detail. "You need to see your dentist to make sure your teeth are healthy enough to take the radiation."

It was 4:00 the Friday before Christmas. We didn't have a dentist. The radiation was to begin January 2. How would we find a dentist willing to take us during the holiday season?

The doctor was unsympathetic and could give us no suggestions of who might take Thom on such short notice. We left the hospital feeling helpless, hopeless and frustrated.

I ranted and raved and cried, "Why didn't they tell us you would need a dental exam? How do they think we can find one now? What dentist is going to take you during the holidays? Oh, what are we going to do?"

Thom didn't say much as he drove home. I felt so sad and mad. I wanted to scream and cry and throw a fit. Then I had this thought, "Pray."

A scripture from the Amplified Bible came to mind, "The earnest (heartfelt, continued) prayer of a righteous man makes tremendous power available-dynamic in its working" (James 5:16).

I began to pray. I was earnest, my prayer was heartfelt. My whole insides seemed to be reaching and crying out to God, "We need a dentist and not just any dentist. We need one that will be extra gentle, one that will not hurt Thom's tongue and mouth. We need an appointment within the next two weeks. Oh God, please help us." Then I prayed in tongues because I didn't know what else to pray.

We were about halfway home and God began to answer my prayer. He brought to my mind a conversation I'd had with one of my customers at the beauty shop. She had been telling me about her dentist that was located next to the Dairy Queen in Lake Wales.

"Thom, one of my ladies at the beauty shop goes to a dentist next to the Dairy Queen in Lake Wales. She told me how wonderful he is. Let's drive over there and see if they are still open. Maybe they could help us."

"It's almost 5:00. No one will be there this late, especially with Christmas on Monday," he answered.

"Oh, come on let's check it out, please. It's not out of the way and besides, what do we have to lose?"

Instead of turning toward home he took the road into town toward the Dairy Queen. Sure enough there was the dentist's office, just as my lady had described. Thom pulled into the parking lot and I jumped out of the car and ran to the door, expecting it to be locked. The door opened and I motioned for Thom to come in.

I could tell they were wrapping it up for the day but they didn't act put out that we were there interrupting their home going. Each one was very kind and caring as we explained our predicament.

The dentist and his wife, who was also his assistant, took Thom right in and examined him then. We were overwhelmed with their understanding and compassion. They explained to us that her father had tongue cancer two years before and how God helped them through many hard times with him. This couple that we had never met gave us the encouragement we so desperately needed along with promises to pray for Thom. Our new dentist gave Thom the okay for radiation.

Only God could have set up our divine dental appointment. Only God could use a place, a dentist's office which had always brought horrible dread and fear to me, to bring the flood of help, kindness and compassion that we felt there. God showed us the reality of James 5:16, "The effective prayer of a righteous man can accomplish much."

God continued to help us through the dreaded radiation. Two doctors prepared us for the worse, making sure we understood how hard this would be on Thom. They said he would be unable to eat because of the terrible sores and left the stomach tube in so he could be nourished. They said he would lose weight, be fatigued and his taste buds and salivary glands would be destroyed. They painted a bleak picture for Thom.

God painted a new picture for us. He took us to Habakkuk 3:3-4 and said, "This is what you can expect, 'My splendor covers the heavens, and the earth is full of My praise. My radiance is like the sunlight; I have rays flashing from My hand, and there is the hiding of My power.'"

Several times that night I woke up compelled to pray for Thom and lay my hands on him. I believed it was God's hands on Thom since God lives in me. I believed it was God's radiance, God's radiation going through Thom's body killing any destructive cancer cells.

A week later, four days before the radiation was to begin God gave us another promise from His Word. "When you walk through the fire, you will not be scorched, nor will the flame burn you. For I am the Lord your God, the holy One of Israel, Your Savior; I have given Egypt as your ransom, Cush and Seba in your place. Since you are precious in My sight, since you are honored and I love you . . . Do not fear, for I am with you" (Isaiah 43:2-5).

Thom went through the radiation surprising his doctors and everyone that knew anything about radiation. He continued to work his normal schedule. He didn't need the stomach tube but ate with little discomfort. He didn't lose weight. He brought joy, laughter and a great testimony to the power of God to all the staff in the radiation department. They were all sad to see him finish because he was such a delight to work with.

What a great God we have! From the beginning of our trial we knew our trust had to be in God. He is trustworthy.

"But I have trusted in Your loving kindness; my heart shall rejoice in Your salvation. I will sing to the Lord, because He has dealt bountifully with me" (Psalm 13:5-6).

Chapter Eight

The next several months were some of the best in our thirty-two years of marriage. Our life returned to normal and it almost seemed like the invasion of cancer had only been a horrible nightmare.

Every appointment with the doctor was positive with no trace of cancer. The feeding tube was removed and Thom was able to eat all the foods he enjoyed, especially steak. His speech showed barely a trace of impediment. We knew the battle had been won. Thom was on earth's side of his win/win situation.

Smoking cigarettes had been a part of Thom's life for forty years. He couldn't seem to give it up until the doctor pronounced, "Its cancer and it was caused by smoking. You need to quit."

Smoking had kept him from doing many things in the church but he made up for all the lost opportunities. He became the spiritual giant I had prayed for. He was voted to serve on the deacon board and worked on the church budget, causing it to operate more efficiently. When the pastor asked him to teach a Wednesday night service he was elated.

Listening to him teaching from the book of James and remembering all he had been through I was bursting with gratitude for what God had done. I was so thankful the battle was over and Thom was on this side of his win/win situation. I wanted to stand up and cheer for God and Thom.

God took care of my dream as He had promised when He told me to help Thom get his dream. I was asked to be on staff as the pastor's assistant. I taught a Sunday morning and Wednesday evening Bible class, started a women's ministry and often filled in for the pastor when he couldn't preach.

Thom and I joined the worship team and eagerly looked forward to Tuesday night practice. We were taught to worship the Lord, to seek Him, to please Him and in doing that we were given a taste of the heavenly realm.

Then on Sunday and Wednesday we were able to share that with the other people.

Using the gifts God had placed within us and truly worshipping Him made our life extremely happy. Our little church was growing. God was using us. Add to that a group of friends that God brought together, well, I knew life couldn't get any better.

Eight months had passed since that dark November day the doctor proclaimed, "Its cancer." We celebrated thirty two years of marriage at our favorite beach resort. Everything seemed so perfect until the day we got home. Trying to be casual Thom showed me a couple small holes under his tongue. He tried to convince me and himself it was from the nuts on a hot fudge sundae we'd had while on our anniversary trip.

Monday couldn't come quick enough for us to schedule a doctor's appointment. When the doctor examined Thom he said it looked like more than an irritation caused by nuts on a sundae. He advised us to go to a well known cancer treatment center in Tampa. When we left his office Thom had an appointment in Tampa the following week.

The sixty mile drive to Tampa was tense. We had no idea what to expect. We both detested going to the doctor and even more the hospital. When the big gray building came in to sight all I could think was, "I do not want to go in there." Even though the day was bright and sunny and the campus beautifully landscaped I was under an ominous cloud of oppression.

We'd been told this was one of the best places for cancer treatment. I tried to catch a thread of hope to cling to. Inside the air felt heavy and sad in spite of the kind and helpful people that greeted us. Extremely sick people seemed to be every where I looked.

The doctor was an older man that gave some comfort by his confident and matter of fact manner. Over shadowing the comfort was a sense of doom that made my stomach sick and my heart break. I felt like I couldn't handle seeing my husband go through this pain again. Our weekly and at times daily visits over the next two years always yielded the same quivering stomach and sad, dull heart ache.

The day was spent getting biopsies, a cat scan, ex-rays and blood work. Finally the doctor gave his verdict. "You need surgery as soon as possible." A date was set and we left planning to return in two weeks.

Thom was relieved and hopeful. He liked his new doctor and enjoyed sharing a fish tale with him and the male nurse that assisted the doctor. I felt sick and wanted to cry my eyes out but that would have to wait until we got home where I would lock myself in the bathroom and let it pour. Thom remained positive and acted lighthearted stopping to enjoy a sandwich and fries on the way home. I choked the food down trying not to show how I really felt.

At home, after a good cry in the bathroom, I went to my quiet spot and grabbed my Bible. "God," I cried, "I've got to hear from You! I need help! I just can't go through this again. Lord, please help!" I started looking at verses I'd underlined, crying between each one.

I came to Philippians 4:6-7 and it seemed like God Himself was saying the words to me, "Be anxious for nothing, but in everything by prayer and supplication with thanksgiving let your requests be made known to God. And the peace of God, which surpasses all comprehension, will guard your hearts and your minds in Christ Jesus."

I thought, "I can do that. I can ask God for what I want for Thom and I can do it with thanksgiving."

I began to ask God to heal Thom, to help us through this. Taking God at His word I did the asking and God gave the peace.

Chapter Nine

Waking up the morning of Thom's surgery I hoped the dread I felt was from a bad dream. I couldn't get rid of the sick feelings in my stomach. I faced the fact that we were indeed going to the hospital and that Thom was to have his second surgery for cancer. I tried to stir up some joy but the longing for my life without cancer was stronger.

The road to Tampa seemed to drag on forever. Instead of trying to make conversation we sang along with our favorite worship tapes. Between songs I asked Thom, "How do people make it through troubles without depending on the Lord for help?"

Before he could answer my question our favorite song began to play. We sang from the depths of our souls, "In Your presence that's where I belong, in Your presence that's where I am strong, seeking Your face, touching Your grace, in Your presence O God."

The heaviness I woke up with and couldn't seem to shake left as we sang to the Lord. By the time we arrived at the cancer center I had regained strength and hope.

Thom was his usual calm self and joked with the nurses preparing him for surgery. As they were getting ready to roll him off to surgery Thom had one request, "Can we pray before I go?"

Again family, friends and pastor were there to pray and encourage me and my daughter, Holly. We sat, we waited, we drank coffee, we prayed. The hours dragged on and each time the phone rang we hoped it would be for us saying the surgery was done and the doctor would be out to talk to us. We were the last ones to get the call. Most of the people had left. It felt like midnight but it was only around seven o'clock.

When the doctor came out he took Holly and I down a long hallway to talk. He explained how the tumor had spread behind Thom's ear and up in to his neck. "I removed as much as possible," he grimly reported, "and I only removed about an inch of his tongue."

I never repeated his grim prognosis. I was determined to believe God's promises for healing. I would hold on to the Word God had spoken to me a year and a half ago, "This sickness is not unto death but for the glory of God" (John 11:4).

Seeing Thom in the recovery room tore my heart apart. How could all this be happening to my vibrant husband? It felt like my life was draining away but I had to smile and be strong for him.

He only wanted to know one thing mouthing the words, "Can I still sing?" He didn't ask, "Did they get it all? Am I going to be okay?"

I had only one answer for him, "Yes, of course you can!"

Everything about the second surgery was more difficult than the first. I stayed with Thom day and night, sharing his hospital room. I had to work hard to keep my peace and often failed. A dark sadness hovered over me. Maybe it was all the seriously and terminally ill patients that filled every room. Maybe it was the threat and fear of death that so often accompanies cancer.

Thom acted peaceful and happy most of the time. I think he was relieved to get help rather than hear, "There is nothing more we can do." He loved to talk and joke around and losing part of his tongue didn't slow him down. He used a dry erase board to share a joke, give praise to God and tell a fish story. He was unable to talk but his communication was as lively as ever.

Two weeks after his surgery we went back for a check up. He had a tube hanging out of his nose, his four front teeth on the top and bottom had been pulled and an inch of his tongue was missing. That didn't stop him from talking to the woman next to him.

She told him about the surgery she needed and how afraid she was. It sounded like the surgery he had done. I thought he was going to try to tell her about his surgery but carefully pronouncing each word he asked, "Do you know Jesus?"

She looked puzzled and I knew she didn't understand what he'd said so I repeated for him, "Do you know Jesus?"

Her sullen face lit up as she shared how Jesus had helped her through her first surgery seven years earlier. She told us about the church she visited and how the pastor had prayed for her. Quietly reflecting for a minute she said, "I know that's why everything went so well back then."

A few minutes before we were called in to see the doctor the three of us held hands and prayed for each other. How simple yet profound to ask a stranger in need, "Do you know Jesus?"

Within a few weeks Thom returned to work. Thom's speech improved and we were ready to get back on the worship team at church. Tuesday night arrived and we almost flew the six miles to church for practice.

Michael, our worship leader, started the evening with time to be quiet before the Lord and prepare our hearts for worship. When we came together to sing it wasn't just a practice. We were there to worship God. We took our places next to the keyboard ready to sing and Michael announced, "I have a new song for us tonight." He played a familiar tune and when he began to sing the words Thom immediately joined in, "In Your presence that's where I belong, in Your presence that's where I am strong, seeking Your face, touching Your grace, in Your presence O God." Thom sang as if he was before the throne singing to God alone. At that moment I knew Thom truly believed he was in a win/win situation.

Chapter Ten

The year following Thom's second surgery we spent much of our time traveling to Tampa for more radiation and check-ups. Highway Sixty became as familiar as the street we lived on. We continued to work our part time jobs, serve at church and live as normally as possible. We had to learn how to cope with our constant intruder, cancer.

Waiting for the results of a biopsy was agony. Several days pondering, "Is it malignant?" Then I'd condemn myself for thinking that way instead of standing strong on the promises of God's healing. I knew I should not allow myself to think malignancy. I knew I should replace my fearful thoughts with the truth of God's Word. I knew all the right things to do. I'd studied faith and taught others how to walk by faith.

I never quit believing that God's Word is the truth. I knew any failure to receive God's promises wasn't because God didn't want to give it to us. The Bible says, "If some did not believe, their unbelief will not nullify the faithfulness of God, will it? May it never be! Rather, let God be found true, though every man be found a liar" (Romans 3:3-4).

The Bible clearly reveals it is always God's will to heal us. Jesus is the "exact representation of His nature" (Hebrews 1:3). Every where Jesus went He healed the sick. I poured over the Gospels putting myself and Thom in the place of each one that received healing.

I tried to identify with the Canaanite woman that chased after Jesus crying out for Him to heal her demon possessed daughter. He seemed to ignore her but she didn't give up. Jesus told her healing was the children's bread and she quickly replied, "Yes, Lord; but even the dogs feed on the crumbs which fall from their master's table." Then Jesus said to her, "O woman, your faith is great; it shall be done for you as you wish." Her daughter was healed at once (Matthew 15:22-28).

Over and over it is recorded how Jesus healed the sick and almost always pointed out that it was their faith that made them well. When He could heal only a few in his home town the Bible says, "And he did not do many miracles there because of their unbelief" (Matthew 15:58).

Thom and I started out strong in faith, holding firm to the promises of God. We experienced many miracles in this battle. No matter what we experienced God never changed, He didn't waver and His will remained the same.

It is always God's will to heal us. Jesus never told anyone, "I'm not going to heal you." The truth is, "He Himself took our infirmities and carried away our diseases" (Matthew 8:17). Jesus took care of the root of sickness, sin. "He Himself bore our sins in His body on the cross, so that we might die to sin and live to righteousness; for by His wounds you were healed" (I Peter 2:24).

Jesus took all of our sin and sickness in His own body over two thousand years ago. Healing belongs to the child of God whether any one receives it or not. Many are not saved from their sins because they choose not to believe in what Jesus did on the cross for them. Many are not healed because they don't know that His death also paid for the healing of their body.

I woke up to sunshine and the familiar sick feeling in my stomach. It had been five days since they took the biopsy. I knew I would have to call that day. "Should I call early or wait until later in the day?" I asked myself. "Am I prolonging the agony unnecessarily? Maybe it will be good news."

I should have been accustomed to the torture. It was the sixth time in two years I had to wait for news of Thom's biopsy. It hadn't gotten any easier with time. Experience had only shown me that I can get through it even though fear tries to smother me with depression.

I decided to call early and get it over with. The news was bad. More treatments, maybe more surgery, what next I wondered?

I felt beat down and weak. I decided to go to the weekly prayer group at church. I couldn't get myself to pray so I listened to everyone else. I began thinking, "Why do we have to go through this?"

My friends were singing songs of praise. I knew I should join them but the words stuck in my throat. It seemed impossible to sing praise that day. Finally I squeaked out the words, "I love You, Lord, and I lift my voice to worship You." With each word I felt strengthened.

I knelt down at the altar. I laid aside my trouble. I focused on Jesus. He began to teach me how to walk above the trials we face in this life.

When I let my troubles bring me down I give that trouble lordship in my life. I replace my Lord Jesus with the trouble, in this case, cancer. Cancer had become the god in my life. I'd allowed it to depress me, condemn me, terrify me and control my every thought, emotion and action.

God revealed to me that I had set Thom above Him. I was more concerned about Thom getting healed than glorifying God and giving Him the praise He created me to give. Jesus said in John 4:23, "But an hour is coming and now is, when the true worshipers will worship the Father in spirit and truth; for such people the Father seeks to be His worshipers."

True worship is surrender. Abraham is an example of true worship. God told him, "Take now your son, your only son, whom you love, Isaac, and go to the land of Moriah, and offer him there as a burnt offering on one of the mountains of which I will tell you" (Genesis 22:2).

When he arrived at the place God told him, Abraham said to the others, "Stay here with the donkey, and I and the lad will go over there; and we will worship and return to you" (Genesis 22:5).

He was going to give his son, his only son, the son he loved as a sacrifice to God. Abraham surrendered what he loved most, he gave him up to God and he called that worship. He was willing to kill his son in obedience to God. He prepared the altar and laid his beloved son on it. He held the knife, ready to plunge it into his son. Abraham called that worship.

Worship is much more than singing songs to God. Worship is giving up all to God, letting go of all that is more important than Him. Worship is surrender to God.

When I surrendered to fear and depression, let it take a hold of me, I was worshipping my troubles rather than God. I let my trouble be my god. Jesus faced this temptation in the wilderness. The devil told him to fall down and worship him and he would give Jesus the kingdoms of this world. Jesus replied to his offer, "Go, Satan! For it is written, YOU SHALL WORSHIP THE LORD YOUR GOD AND SERVE HIM ONLY" (Matthew 4:10).

The devil continues to throw that same temptation at me disguised as fear, depression, discouragement, condemnation, and doubt. When I surrender to those things they become my god. In reality I am worshipping or surrendering to the devil. I take Jesus off the throne of my heart and put Satan in His place.

When I saw the truth of what I was doing by surrendering to my troubles and letting fear and sadness control me I determined to change. I made the decision to worship the Lord at all times. I would keep my mind on Him and praise Him. I often failed but each time I did I practiced I John 1:9, "If we confess our sins, He is faithful and righteous to forgive us our sins and to cleanse us from all unrighteousness."

Chapter Eleven

"Its cancer," the doctor stated. I looked at Thom listening to the words that had been pronounced over him for the fourth time in a year and a half. He appeared so calm except for the slight twitch in his hands.

"How can he be so calm?" I thought to myself. I felt like screaming and kicking everyone in sight, especially the doctor. My stomach felt like it had been punched a dozen times and my head was pounding.

Thom and the doctor were discussing his third surgery so unruffled and coolly.

They could have been planning a fishing trip except they were using words like reconstruction, tracheotomy, swelling and speech difficulty.

Another conversation was going on in my head. "Why do we have to go through this again, Lord?" I didn't give Him time to answer before I shot several more questions at Him. "What about all the promises in the Bible for healing? What is the problem here? What are we doing wrong? Why isn't he healed?"

All I heard in response to my desperate questioning was, "My Word has not changed and I have not changed."

On the way home Thom continued to be calm, joking and making plans for his surgery that had been scheduled in two weeks. We stopped for lunch but it was hard to get the food down. I had to keep holding back the tears I didn't want Thom to see.

Back in the car I continued my conversation with God, questions popping up right and left. In the middle of, "Why don't You . . ." He gently reminded me of Psalm 9.

Only six hours earlier, before leaving home for the appointment I had read Psalm 9:1-2. I was excited as I promised God I'd do the four "I wills." I had been determined to make them my way of life from then on. I truly wanted to live for God and please Him; this was how I could do that.

A few minutes after making my promise the phone rang. It was my daughter twelve hundred miles away. After a quick, "Hi, Mom, "she hesitantly said, "I think God gave me a word today for you and Dad. When I was praying I felt like I was to tell you to read Psalm 9."

All I could say was, "You are right on. God gave me the same direction just a few minutes ago. Thank you for stepping out and obeying God. I will share this with your Dad. Thanks, Heather, I love you."

I shared with Thom the four "I wills" that God had given us in Psalm 9:1-2.

"I WILL GIVE THANKS TO THE LORD WITH ALL MY HEART;
I WILL TELL OF ALL YOUR WONDERS.
I WILL BE GLAD AND EXULT IN YOU;
I WILL SING PRAISE TO YOUR NAME, O MOST HIGH."

How could I have let a bad report from the doctor cancel out the plan God had given me a few hours earlier? I was embarrassed remembering how determined I had been to do it and then so easily forgot my promise.

"Lord, please forgive me. I'm so sorry for letting fear and doubt take control of me. I promised You I'd do the four "I wills" in Psalm nine and I've acted like You left town. Please help me."

I felt the Lord loving me with these words, "This battle with cancer isn't about living or dying. It is about giving thanks to Me with all your heart even when the report is not what you wanted to hear. It is about telling of My wonders in the middle of the battle. It is about being glad and exulting in Me when you want to scream and cry. It is about singing praises to My name when it looks like things are getting worse. It is about touching My grace to rise above the battle you face."

We had many opportunities to be mad at God, question His love for us and even walk away from Him. People often do. I had a friend that lost her husband to cancer after watching him suffer for several years. For ten years after he died she refused to continue her relationship with God and go to church. She felt she had every right to be angry with God because of all the pain her husband had experienced even though she constantly prayed for him.

Life on this earth can be difficult. Cinderella endings don't always happen. The hard times can seem monumental. We often allow ourselves to be crushed and controlled by the struggles we have.

Bad times feel like they last forever and we tend to get lost in a tunnel of darkness. The Bible says in James 4:14, "Yet you do not know what your life will be like tomorrow. You are just a vapor that appears for a little while and then vanishes away." Breathe on a mirror and watch how quickly the vapor disappears. That is how fast our life on earth is.

We are told in Colossians 3:2, "Set your mind on the things above, not on the things that are on earth." Each time we heard bad news about Thom's health we had a choice to make. We could focus on things here or things above. God revealed Psalm nine to our family to help us focus on the things above.

Each time I gave thanks to the Lord with all my heart I touched God's grace. When I would tell of His wonders I would enter in to God's grace. Choosing to be glad and exult in God brought a new flow of God's grace. Singing praise to His name not only touched God's grace but also His face.

God did not tell me to give thanks for the cancer that was trying to destroy my husband because that would oppose the will of God. "He is our healer" (Exodus 15:26). God sent Jesus to give us abundant life (John 10:10), to take sickness away (Matthew 8:17) and to release us from the curse (Galatians 3:13).

Everywhere Jesus went He healed the people. He never told them to thank God for their sickness. Sickness never brought glory to God. Studying the gospels I found that God is glorified when people are healed and set free.

"In everything give thanks; for this is God's will for you in Christ Jesus" (I Thessalonians 5:18). Notice it doesn't say for everything but in everything. While we are in the battle we are to give thanks to God for Who He is and all He has done. Thom and I didn't do well obeying this command. We usually were overwhelmed by the doctor's report and by the symptoms we saw. We let our emotions dictate our response.

Giving thanks to God magnifies Him rather than the problem. Psalm 69:29-31 says, "But I am afflicted and in pain; may Your salvation, O God, set me securely on high, I will praise the name of God with song and magnify Him with thanksgiving. And it will please the Lord better than an ox or a young bull with horns and hoofs."

God never stopped loving us or withheld His grace because we failed to respond with praise. He knows us and He loves us and He never leaves us. He meets us where our faith is. Thom's faith was in the truth that he was in a win/win situation. He believed that if he lived or died he was a winner. How could it be losing if he died and went to heaven? Isn't that what all Christians are looking forward to?

Chapter Twelve

I tried to get comfortable in the reclining chair I'd pulled up next to Thom's hospital bed. My right hand went through the side rail holding his hand. My left arm clutched the big pink pillow I'd brought from home. My eyes settled on the stuffed cat cuddled up next to Thom.

The day before, after Thom's two and a half hour surgery he made motions of petting his beloved cat, Molly. Later I saw the stuffed, long-haired cat in the hospital gift shop. It looked so real I had to get it for Thom. I was always looking for ways to bring a smile to his face that was getting distorted with each surgery. Everyone that came into the room commented on the cat, several thought it was alive. I loved seeing Thom smile as I told them about his cat.

While Thom slept I was hit with the thought that the stuffed cat was much more than a smile collector. I thought back to the month before when Molly was very sick. At first the vet thought Molly had pneumonia but as she grew worse she was tested for leukemia.

Waiting anxiously to hear the results of the blood test I prayed for the gray and white Persian that my husband adored. I felt anger rising up as I thought about how heartbroken Thom would be if Molly died. Accompanying my anger was a desire to fight. Like thunder clouds rolling in before a storm the Word of God came rushing to my mind preparing me for battle.

I remembered Jesus saying in Luke 10:19, "Behold, I have given you authority to tread upon serpents and scorpions, and over all the power of the enemy, and nothing shall injure you." If Molly died Thom would be injured.

I took the sword of the Spirit and went after the serpent that was trying to kill our cat. I shouted, "No, devil! You aren't going to kill Molly! I tread on you! I'm finished letting you tread on me and my family, causing one injury after another! You leave Molly, take your sickness and go!"

I continued to shout the Scriptures that were filling my mind. With each one I felt more power and authority rise up inside of me. I took my stand and refused to let the devil win.

It couldn't have been more than ten minutes and I felt I needed to go to the animal hospital. I took the bottle of anointing oil and hurried over before their noon closing. "I've got to see my cat, Molly," I said as I rushed in.

The receptionist led me back to Molly's cage. I dabbed oil on my hands and picked up my sickly cat. I softly but firmly commanded, "Sickness leave this cat now in Jesus name." I cuddled Molly and whispered in her ear, "Molly, you be healed." My mission was accomplished. I put Molly back in her cage and left.

Three hours later I heard from the vet. She reported, "Molly's fever broke and is eating and acts much better." We brought the cat home the next day and blood tests showed no leukemia.

Reliving my battle for Molly's healing the stuffed cat reminded me I must do the same with the cancer that was trying to take Thom's life. I had grown weary and felt badly beaten by so many bad reports. I had not been consistent in using the power and authority that belonged to me.

We have an enemy, the devil. He came to steal, kill and destroy (John 10:10). His goal is to steal the Word of God out of our heart so that we will not believe and be saved and healed (Luke 8:12). In a parable Jesus tells of four people that hear the Word. Only one out of those four bear fruit or receives what God has for him. In Mark four Jesus explains that those that do receive from God get thirty, sixty or a hundred-fold.

Look at the numbers. Only one out of four that hears God's Word believes and receives. If you put all those that receive in a group only one out of three receives the whole thing or one hundred percent. Luke 8:15 tells us, "But the seed in the good soil, these are the ones who have heard the word in an honest and good heart, and hold it fast, and bear fruit with perseverance." When things get tough we often let go of what we believe in God's Word. We don't use the perseverance called for in many situations. Like Jesus explained in this same parable, "we believe for awhile, and in time of temptation fall away" (Luke 8:13).

Jairus came to Jesus to heal his daughter that was dying. On the way to his house someone came and told Jairus to forget it, his daughter had died. "But when Jesus heard this, He answered him, 'Do not be afraid any longer; only believe, and she will be made well'" (Luke 8:50). Thom and I became afraid many times and believed more in what we could see and what the doctors told us than in what the Word of God had to say about God's provision for healing.

If the devil can steal God's Word out of our heart our faith stops working. "Faith comes from hearing and hearing by the Word of Christ" (Romans 10:17). When the disciples failed to set free a demon possessed boy they asked Jesus, "Why couldn't we set him free?" Jesus told them plainly, "Because of the littleness of your faith, for truly I say to you, if you have faith the size of a mustard seed, you will say to this mountain, 'Move from here to there,' and it will move; and nothing will be impossible to you" (Matthew 17:20).

We are warned in I Peter 5:8-9, "Be of sober spirit, be on the alert. Your adversary, the devil, prowls around like a roaring lion, seeking someone to devour. But resist him, firm in your faith, knowing that the same experiences of suffering are being accomplished by your brethren who are in the world."

Paul gives specific directions for standing up against the devil and overcoming his plans to destroy us. "Finally, be strong in the Lord and in the strength of His might. Put on the full armor of God, so that you will be able to stand firm against the schemes of the devil. For our struggle is not against flesh and blood, but against the rulers, against the powers, against the world forces of this darkness, against the spiritual forces of wickedness in the heavenly places. Therefore, take up the full armor of God, so that you will be able to resist in the evil day, having done everything, to stand firm, having girded your loins with truth, and having put on the breastplate of righteousness, and having shod your feet with the preparation of the gospel of peace; in addition to all, taking up the shield of faith with which you will be able to extinguish all the flaming arrows of the evil one. And take the helmet of salvation, and the sword of the Spirit, which is the word of God" (Ephesians 6:10-17).

Each piece of the armor protects our faith. The shield we hold out in front of us is faith, it stops all the lies the devil throws at us. We can chop up the devil with our sword, the word of God that we speak.

Jesus defeated the devil! Hebrews 2:14 says, "He rendered powerless him who had the power of death, that is, the devil."

Jesus removed everything the devil could use against us. He removed the power of sin, guilt, shame and condemnation. "When you were dead in your transgressions and the uncircumcision of your flesh, He made you alive together with Him, having forgiven us all our transgressions, having canceled out the certificate of debt consisting of decrees against us, which was hostile to us; and He has taken it out of the way, having nailed it to the cross. When

He disarmed the rulers and authorities, He made a public display of them, having triumphed over them through Him" (Colossians 2:13-15).

Jesus gave us His name and His authority to use against the devil. "The seventy returned with joy, saying, "Lord, even the demons are subject to us in Your name." And He said to them, "I was watching Satan fall from heaven like lightening. Behold, I have given you authority to tread on serpents and scorpions, and over all the power of the enemy, and nothing will injure you" (Luke 10:17-19).

Jesus gave His life and shed His blood to give us power over the enemy, the devil. "And the great dragon was thrown down, the serpent of old who is called the devil and Satan, who deceives the whole world; he was thrown down to the earth, and his angels with him. And they overcame him because of the blood of the Lamb and because of the word of their testimony, and they did not love their life even when faced with death" (Revelations 12:9,11).

God has given us everything we need to overcome the devil. God wants us healed and whole. He is a good God and His will for us is always abundant life.

With God there are no failures. He meets us where we are and "He always leads us in triumph in Christ" (II Corinthians 2:14). That is why Thom could say with great faith, "I'm in a win/win situation."

Chapter Thirteen

After Thom's third surgery I had to learn some basic nursing skills. The removal of the tracheotomy tube left an open wound in his neck and the new feeding tube placed directly in his stomach needed special care. I had to do things I thought I didn't have the stamina for. I had to change my thinking from, "I can't do that," to "If Thom needs it done I will do it and God will help me." So I did do those things and God did help me.

Several weeks later Thom was feeling strong. He was ready to go back to work at the golf shop he so dearly loved. His neck was healed with no evidence of the tracheotomy. He still had the stomach tube but by tucking it in his pants and covering it with his shirt no one would know it was there. His speech was difficult to understand but he worked hard at trying to pronounce each word clearly. He wouldn't give up trying to communicate and often wrote what he couldn't get out clearly enough.

Winter golf season was about to begin. Thom made an appointment with his boss to talk about coming back to his job. Work had always been an important part of his life. He loved his job at the golf shop. He had developed good relationships with the people he served and he cared deeply for them.

When he returned from the meeting I could tell it hadn't been good. I didn't realize how badly it had affected Thom until later. He tried to tell me what happened but all he could say was, "I can never go back to work in the golf shop. My speech is too hard to understand. I cried right there in front of my boss."

Even though that happened several years ago I can still feel the pain he carried home that day. Winter in Florida is glorious but it wasn't glorious at our house that year. My normally happy and humorous husband was sad, quiet and depressed. I'd never seen him like that. I prayed. I tried to do things to brighten his days but nothing brought his joy back.

Watching him sink deeper into darkness I had to get help for him. I knew he'd be upset with me but I told the doctor I was very concerned about Thom's depression. Medication and counseling was the doctor's solution. I didn't see much improvement but I hoped the daily dose of anti-depressant was easing his mental and emotional pain.

Thom's time was spent in the living room, a permanent part of the bright flowered couch, watching television during the day, sleeping at night. He no longer cared about fishing. Visitors were few. The man I'd spent over thirty years with was gone, replaced by a sick and tired victim of cancer.

Over the years I've questioned God, "Why wasn't Thom healed? What happened?" We both knew what the Bible taught about healing. We knew that God provided healing through His son Jesus Christ. We had experienced God's healing power many times. He always answered my question the same way, "Thom gave up the day he lost his job."

Losing his job destroyed his hope for the future. The Bible says, "Hope deferred makes the heart sick, but desire fulfilled is a tree of life" (Proverbs 13:12). When Thom lost his job his heart was broken. He was heartsick.

"Faith is the evidence of things hoped for," according to Hebrews 11:1. When he lost his hope his faith diminished.

Thom's job defined who he was. The thirty years he worked for General Motors he called himself a factory rat. I hated that he saw himself that way. It wasn't the right name for a man that provided so well for his family and always did what he felt was best for us.

Working at the golf shop for three years he received a new picture of himself. He no longer referred to himself as a factory rat. He was happy, fulfilled and respected by all who knew him. He gave of himself and shared his love for Jesus. The people there shared their lives with him. He had found his place to shine. When the job was over his light went out.

I received this note from one of the ladies he helped: "Thom planted a few pineapple tops for me and one grew in the perfect spot. Nature met all of its needs. I have thought of it as a prayer pineapple as each time I walk near it I have lifted Thom up to the Lord. Now it's like a living monument to Thom.

We'll never know the actual number of living monuments Thom's faith and testimony inspired. His life was a garden of praise to the Lord's glory-always growing and in full bloom. He met each surgical complication with amazing grace. His love for the Lord never weakened.

Thom may now be absent from the world but we know his life was used for the fullest and is now glorified. I send you my admiration for Thom as a bouquet. May its fragrance wrap you and your family in peace and love."

Even though Thom lost his hope for his future here on earth he never lost his hope for heaven. The following year his hope was to be with Jesus. One day he wrote to me, "I want to go home." I wrote back, "You are home." He responded, "Home with Jesus."

He never stopped believing he was in a win/win situation. The win he wanted after two years of standing strong in faith and believing to be healed changed to a desire to go to his home in heaven. Thom believed as Paul did in Philippians 1:23, "Having the desire to depart and be with Christ, for that is very much better."

Chapter Fourteen

The first two years dealing with cancer were extremely difficult even though God always met us at the point of our faith. Standing firm on His promises brought the victory each time and we experienced many miracles. The third year turned in to a horrendous nightmare. Thom gave up and cancer ravaged his body.

Support from church and friends dwindled. One day I was crying to my friend Robin, "Where is everyone? Doesn't anyone care?" When I shared our needs she heard my despair. From then on she and her family were there for us and helped us face every challenge.

Robin brought to us joy and laughter along with her strong faith in God. She was sensitive to our weaknesses, knew what we needed and always made us laugh. Everyone needs a Robin in their life especially when facing the tough times.

My parents moved to Florida to be near us a year after we moved down. Dad had been taking care of my mother for several years. She was completely disabled after a stroke and heart surgery. My father did everything for her so I tried to be of help to him when I could but as Thom got worse it became harder for me to be there as much as I wanted.

After a severe blood infection the doctor recommended a nursing home for my mother. She hated it and I was determined to get her out and back to her home. Again God sent the right person to help us, Juanita. With her help my mother was able to come back home.

For several months I'd been concerned about my father. He didn't seem to be thinking right and often got mixed up. The receptionist at the doctor's office told me Dad had come in for an appointment he didn't have. She said he went out to the car and came back and repeated the same conversation. I knew then I wasn't imagining his strange behavior.

Not only was he having memory problems but physical difficulties had come up. A colonoscopy and biopsy showed he had colon cancer. The doctor scheduled him for surgery. I tried not to panic trying to figure out how to care for my mother while Dad was in the hospital and take care of Thom.

As always God had everything under control. When I told Juanita our dilemma she immediately responded, "I'll stay with Mrs. Johnson as long as you need me to. Don't be concerned." That day she quit her job with the local nursing agency and prepared to stay at my parent's home.

I was bombarded with so many thoughts and emotions as I drove home that day. I tried to push them away and focus on the goodness of God. Turning onto my street a wave of panic hit me when I saw an ambulance parked in my driveway.

I rushed in to find Thom hooked up to oxygen. The paramedic explained that Thom had called 911 unable to breathe and they traced the call and came out.

At the hospital a permanent tracheotomy tube was put in and Thom began a hellish round of chemotherapy. I thought I had all the trouble I could tolerate but more was on the way. I lived Psalm 34:19, "Many are the afflictions of the righteous, but the Lord delivers him out of them all."

Dad's surgery went well but when the anesthetic wore off the man I'd known as my Dad was gone. He pulled tubes out and bandages off. Everyday he told of the adventures he'd just returned from. I heard details of a party with the queen of England, hitchhiking to Colorado and hiding in the tunnels beneath the hospital.

One night he called me at 3:00 a.m. demanding, "Come over here right now! I just saw someone get murdered." Trying to convince him that he must have had a bad dream only agitated him more and he hung up on me.

A few minutes later a nurse called saying, "Your father has barricaded himself in his room and we can't calm him down. Would you talk to him on the phone and get him to let us in?" I was unsuccessful. He kept them out for the next two hours. I was unable to leave Thom alone so that I could try to settle my Dad down.

It didn't look like Dad was going to go home and take up his life where he'd left off. Caring for my mother was a big issue. How long would Juanita be willing to stay? Could my parent's afford to pay for Dad's nursing home care and Ma's fulltime care at home?

The questions were answered when my mother passed away a month after Dad's surgery. She had been getting weaker, her body worn out and her heart broken with Dad being away from her so long. As she lay in the hospital bed trying to talk I could barely make out her last words, "Where is Dad? Is Dad dead?"

Even though he had an infection, MRSA, and hospital rules forbid him from entering another part of the hospital, I insisted they bring him to my mother immediately. She was dying and needed to say good bye to her husband of fifty three years. Fifteen minutes later he was sitting beside her bed holding her hand. No words were exchanged, only looks of love. That night my mother died.

The next six months brought more pain than I thought possible. My sweet mother that I loved dearly was gone. My strong, authoritative father had become like the child and I had to be the strong one planning his life and taking care of his personal business. Cancer was destroying more of my husband and the doctors were talking, "Hospice."

God, always my loving Father, gave me what I needed when I needed it. He opened my eyes to what really mattered in this life on earth. I still cried and asked Him, "Why?" I still got angry and questioned, "Where are You?" He still loved me and brought me to His word, the Bible, for my answers.

Questions bombarded my mind regularly. At first I let them stay and entertained them. A party full of tears, self pity and anger would soon be in full swing. Tough times dredge up all kinds of questions.

As time went on I learned not to ask the questions out of anger. Who was I to question angrily the Most High God? How dare I be disrespectful to my Creator. I thought about what God said to Job in chapters thirty eight through forty one. God questioned Job about who made the infinite marvels of nature.

Job answered God," I know You can do all things, and that no purpose of Yours can be thwarted. Who is this that hides counsel without knowledge? Therefore I have declared that which I did not understand, things too wonderful for me, which I do not know. Hear, now, and I will speak; I will ask You, and You instruct me. I have heard of You by the hearing ear; but now my eyes see You; therefore I retract, and repent in dust and ashes" (Job 42:1-6).

God wants to answer our questions. The key to hearing the answers is the condition of our heart. Am I asking God because I'm sad and mad and can't understand why He is letting such horrible things happen to me? Or am I humble before Him and ask from a heart that wants to please God, live for Him and glorify Him? The question is, "Who am I living for, me or God?"

Isaiah 45:9-12 deals with the issue of questioning God. "Woe to the one who quarrels with his Maker-an earthenware vessel among the vessels of earth!

Will the clay say to the potter, 'What are you doing?' Or the thing you are making say, 'He has no hands'? Woe to him who says to a father, 'What are you begetting?' Or to a woman, 'To what are you giving birth.'" This scripture shows a disrespectful attitude toward God, one I sometimes slipped in to.

Reading on we are shown how a humble child of God can question the Father. "Thus says the Lord, the Holy One of Israel, and his Maker: 'Ask Me about the things to come concerning My sons, and you shall commit to Me the work of My hands. It is I who made the earth, and created man upon it. I stretched out the heavens with My hands and I ordained all their host.'"

If we have been born again God is our Father. We must give Him the same kind of respect we give our earthly fathers. My Dad would not allow me to speak disrespectfully to him. He could tell my bad attitude by the look on my face, before I said a word he knew I was coming against his authority. He would stop it immediately. My Dad demanded that I treat him with respect. He only let me talk when my heart was soft, then I could ask whatever I needed to know. God, our heavenly Father calls for the same kind of respect. The Bible calls it the fear of the Lord.

I had to make myself stop the angry questioning and say, "God, I trust You. I commit all to You. Please show me what I need to know." I had to stop feeding my need to be the victim, always crying, "poor me."

I had to hook up with Thom and believe with him that we were in a win/win situation. I had to choose to believe whether we live or die we are in a win/win situation. Whether we are sick or healthy we win, whether we are rich or poor we win, no matter what goes on around us we win. God's promise had to become mine, "But thanks be to God, who always leads us in triumph in Christ and manifests through us the sweet aroma of the knowledge of Him in every place" (II Corinthians 2:14).

Life was not the way I would have liked it to be but God showed up at some unexpected times and places and I wouldn't trade that for any story book life. Like the warm fall day a couple months after my mother died when my Dad and I shared the most important moment of his life.

He seemed like his old self that day, quiet and sensible. We started talking about spiritual things which had always been a touchy subject for us. For twenty years I had tried to share with him his need to accept Jesus Christ as his Savior. His reply was always the same, "That's great for you but I don't need that."

That day was different. I told him that we all sin, that we all need God's forgiveness (Romans 3:23). I told him that we deserve to die for our sins but instead Jesus died on the cross and took the punishment for our sin so that we could be forgiven and go to Heaven when we die (Romans 6:23). I explained that we must believe in our heart that Jesus died for our sins and that God raised Him from the dead and we will be saved (Romans 10:8-10).

I asked my Dad, "Would you like to pray and ask God to forgive you and tell Him that you do believe Jesus died for your sins and that He raised Jesus from the dead for you?"

My Dad was a very strong person and no one could ever intimidate him or make him do anything he didn't want to do. When he answered my question with an emphatic, "Yes," I knew he meant business. We prayed a simple prayer that lovely fall day in Florida. I no longer had to hope and pray that my Dad would be saved, I know he is and that I will see him in heaven. I think he will be one of the first to greet me when I get there.

Chapter Fifteen

Making decisions, oh how I hated the responsibility. One of the hardest I ever had to make was in regards to Thom's care; should we have Hospice? Hospice, to me, spelled death. I thought it meant giving up. I knew the care he would get from Hospice would be so much better for him. No more long hours in the hospital emergency rooms laying on a hard, cold table and no more aggressive treatments that took more life out of him than it gave.

Even harder than making the decision to get Hospice care was telling Thom. I hoped I wouldn't have to tell him, that they would come and care for him and he would never know they were from Hospice. They insisted he know so I had to tell him. I think that was the hardest thing I've ever had to do.

Chemotherapy had damaged Thom's hearing. I had to write all our communication as he had been doing since losing so much of his tongue and couldn't talk. Thom's health insurance was changing that month so I tried to make it sound as if we were getting Hospice because of that. I couldn't fool him. His written reply after my explanation was, "Am I dying?"

I couldn't say, "Yes." I wrote on and on about hope, miracles and trusting God. Mostly I cried.

Hospice care would focus on Thom's and my comfort. After three years of struggling with the destruction of cancer we needed comfort and help for our body, soul and spirit. The care givers from Hospice seemed like a troop of angels sent directly from heaven.

Hospice took care of Thom for fifty days. During that time I questioned what the promise meant that God had given me months before Thom was diagnosed with cancer.

"This sickness is not unto death but for the glory of God" (John 11:4). Watching his motionless body wither away looked like this sickness was unto death. What is death? Death means to be separated from God.

When Lazarus died Jesus told his grieving sister, "I am the resurrection and the life; he who believes in Me will live even if he dies, and everyone who lives and believes in Me will never die. Do you believe this" (John 11:25-26)?

How can that be that if we live and believe we will never die? The believer is never separated from God. We are a spirit that lives in a body. Our spirit lives forever, either in heaven or hell, depending on our decision to receive Jesus as Lord and Savior or rejecting Him.

Dying isn't the end for the believer in Jesus Christ. Dying is as simple as stepping out of our fleshly body. Thom stepped out of his body that had been battered and mutilated by cancer and took on the image of the heavenly according to I Corinthians 15:49. "His body was sown a perishable body, it was raised an imperishable body; it was sown in dishonor, it was raised in glory; it was sown in weakness, it was raised in power; it was sown a natural body; it was raised a spiritual body."

Thom's sickness was not unto death! He is seeing the sights of heaven, hearing the music of angels, dancing and shouting for joy in the presence of the Lord. A few days before Thom died the Lord showed me this picture of what Thom would enter into, "Then the eyes of the blind will be opened and the ears of the deaf will be unstopped. Then the lame will leap like a deer, and the tongue of the mute will shout for joy" (Isaiah 35:5-6).

Jesus talked to His disciples about their priorities in Luke 10. They had returned from a powerful time of ministry. People had been healed and set free. They were excitedly telling Jesus, "Lord, even the demons are subject to us in Your name" (Luke 10:17). Jesus told them, "I was watching Satan fall from heaven like lightning. Behold, I have given you authority to tread on serpents and scorpions, and over all the power of the enemy, and nothing will injure you" (Luke 10:18-19). As wonderful as all that is Jesus tells them there is something even better to get excited about. "Nevertheless do not rejoice in this, that the spirits are subject to you, but rejoice that your names are recorded in heaven" (Luke 10:20).

God was saying to me that rather than be sad about Thom not receiving a miracle healing I needed to rejoice that his name was recorded in heaven. Our life on earth is so minute compared to eternity. We get so caught up in our troubles here on earth and often forget that we are just passing through, on our way to a place that has no pain or sorrow, heaven.

Jesus reminded his disciples to rejoice that their names were recorded in heaven. Is your name recorded in heaven? If you aren't certain you need to choose to believe God's Word and act on it now. Accept the fact that you are a sinner that needs a Savior, "For all have sinned and fall short of the glory of God" (Romans 3:23). Realize your sin needs to be dealt with, "For the wages of sin is death, but the free gift of God is eternal life in Christ Jesus our Lord" (Romans 6:23). Know that God has provided a simple way for you to get your name recorded in heaven, "If you confess with your mouth Jesus as Lord, and believe in your heart that God raised Him from the dead, you will be saved" (Romans 10:9).

You can pray this prayer and be born again, become a child of God and know that your name is recorded in heaven. You can know that when your body dies you will go to heaven. "Dear Lord, I confess to You that I have sinned. I ask You to forgive my sins. I believe in my heart that Jesus died on the cross, that he was punished for my sins and that You, God, raised Jesus from the dead so that I could have a new life with You, forgiven and set free from the bondage of my sins. I give myself to You and ask You to make my life pleasing to You. Thank you that my name is recorded in heaven, I rejoice in that. In Jesus' name I pray, Amen."

Thom went home January 19, 2001 at 2:00 a.m. I was sleeping on the couch pulled up next to his hospital bed in the living room of our dream house. I believe the angel that escorted him to heaven touched me on the shoulder on their way out. I woke up listening for his breathing even though I knew he was gone.

The next few days passed quickly with lots of activity and little time to think. I preached his funeral service in Florida. I knew he'd like that. He had always been so proud of my ministry and insisted on using my "reverend" title whenever he could in spite of my protests.

My daughter and I flew to Michigan for another service and burial. Within a week I bought a house and began making plans to move back to Michigan.

Even though I was busy getting ready for my move I had plenty of time to think and cry. Everything reminded me of Thom. Selling his fishing boat was especially hard but I was comforted when a neighbor bought it.

I spent a lot of time reading my Bible and often found written next to verses my prayers for Thom. God answered every one, not always in the way I wanted. My vision had been so limited.

When Jesus was getting ready to leave the earth and go back to heaven He comforted the disciples with these words from John 14:1-3, "Do not let your heart be troubled; believe in God, believe also in Me. In My Father's house are many dwelling places; if it were not so, I would have told you; for I go to prepare a place for you. If I go and prepare a place for you, I will come again and receive you to Myself, that where I am, there you may be also."

Thom has a place there, where Jesus is, a real place. I wanted to see that Thom was happy, that he was okay. I asked the Lord if He would give me a dream of Thom in heaven. I waited and I prayed and nothing came until Easter morning.

I went to church with my daughter, Holly. A play, "Heaven's Gates, Hell's Flames" was being presented. I'd seen it several times in different churches so I knew what to expect. But God had a surprise for me, the answer to my plea, "Let me see Thom in heaven."

The story is about several different people that die and face God after having an opportunity to receive Jesus as their Savior. The ones that chose not to accept Jesus are thrown in to the life-like flames of hell. Those that accepted Jesus are escorted into heaven.

One of the last performers came out, a man that looked identical to Thom when he was in his late twenties, mustache and all. He accepted Jesus as his Savior and was then killed in a car crash. His entrance into heaven was the most glorious of all the actors. He sang the same song that was sung at Thom's funeral in Michigan. It was about getting to heaven and seeing Abraham and all the others. He is so thrilled to be there but he wants to see Jesus, the One Who died for him. The man was so much like Thom, dancing and full of the same kind of enthusiasm he always had. If I didn't know better I would have thought it truly was Thom dancing and singing on that stage.

Only God knew how much I needed to see the scene that represented Thom's new life in the place He had prepared for him. It helped dim the sad pictures of Thom that I had been carrying in my mind.

God answered my prayer on Easter day and I could boldly and confidently say, "cancer can't win! Cancer didn't win!"

www.ingramcontent.com/pod-product-compliance
Lightning Source LLC
Chambersburg PA
CBHW021257280526
45784CB00005B/2406